How to Get Pregnant

How To Boost Your Fertility
For First Time Mom or Dad To Be

Karen Kennedy

PUBLISHED BY:
Karen Kennedy

Disclaimer

The information contained in this book is for general information purposes only. The information is provided by the authors and while we endeavor to keep the information up to date and correct, we make no representations or warranties of any kind, express or implied, about the completeness, accuracy, reliability, suitability or availability with respect to the book or the information, products, services, or related graphics contained in the book for any purpose. Any reliance you place on such information is therefore strictly at your own risk.

TABLE OF CONTENTS

Chapter 1: Introduction

Things to Consider Before Conception

Before you decide to start trying to conceive, there are several things that need to be considered and discussed with your partner. Are you financially secure, physically and emotionally healthy, and is your relationship healthy? Do you have friends with babies? If not, you may notice some changes in how you interact with childless friends. Are your living arrangements the right choice for a child? Will a baby fit into your life plan?

Financial Security: While financial security isn't a definite must when deciding if it is the right time to try for a baby, it is helpful and should be considered. It is nice to be able to afford the things you want for your baby and yourself, to know that you can provide for their future, as well as for their present. However, for some people financial security may seem impossible and waiting for that moment can mean that they will never have a child. If you are not financially secure, there may be some things you can do to ensure that you have some money set aside before the baby is born. Start a savings account and stop spending money on luxury items. That means no more five dollar coffees, no more dinners out every week, no more name-brand items. Have enough money saved in your account to be able to pay your bills for at least six months in case you lose your job or are laid off. Unfortunately, being laid off is something that happens often and cannot be forecast in enough time to ensure your stability. For instance, when we decided to have a second child, my husband had a wonderful job; we were financially secure, and felt it was the right time to conceive. Two months after conception, we found out he was going to be laid off after the baby was born. So while we started the pregnancy feeling safe and secure, we ended it not knowing when and if either of us would find work. We were still able to raise a happy, healthy child, despite whatever hardships we may have faced. Hopefully, you will have the support of friends or family if you need it.

However, babies can get expensive. There's always a way to cut costs by not purchasing the latest, high-end baby gear, but even things like diapers can add up quickly over the months. If you have a restricted budget, this could be an issue for you. Decide early on, even before conception, if you would consider breastfeeding. Not only is this the best choice for your baby's health, but it is also budget friendly. A can of formula may cost upwards of 13 dollars, and you will go through more than four cans of formula a month. Breastfeeding is an instant way to save money. Another way to save money is to decide if you are going to use disposable diapers or cloth diapers. While the initial purchase of cloth diapers can exceed 100 dollars (or more), in the end, you wind up saving thousands of dollars, especially if you use the diapers for more than one child. It is never too early to start educating yourself on ways to save money on baby products.

Emotional Health: Are you emotionally ready to have a baby? If you still feel like you want to go to parties, hang out with friends, or play video games all the time, you may not be in an emotional state that is optimal for a baby. Another thing to consider is how you are emotionally, not just on the "I want to have fun" front, but also psychologically. If you aren't emotionally mature now, you won't suddenly become so once the baby is born. Babies create a lot of work and sleepless nights. Emotional health is important for a healthy pregnancy, as well as for a healthy life for the baby. Babies need you there for them when they are born, they don't need caregivers; they need mommies. If you plan on going out a lot after the baby is born, you may wish to wait a bit until you are able to put the baby first.

Relationship Status: It is also important to review your relationship. You and your partner are the core of the family unit. With a weak foundation, you will only be setting yourselves up for failure. A baby is not a solution to any problem. Make sure you are capable of working together as a team before bringing in a new factor. One of the questions your caregiver will ask you is if you feel like you are in danger from physical or emotional abuse at home. They ask that question to ensure your well-being as well as that of the child's. You cannot have a healthy pregnancy if you are constantly abused, hurt, or stressed. So, if you fight often, feel belittled, or feel endangered, it isn't the right time for you to conceive a child. You are thinking about bringing a new life into the mix, and if you aren't safe, your child won't be safe.

Childless Friends: Do any of your friends have babies or will you be the first? Be realistic and realize that a baby will affect your Saturday nights. It may take some getting used to for your baby-less friends, but hopefully they will adjust to the new swing of things. If you have friends who have babies, however, they will be a great source for help, ideas, and baby play dates. When you have friends who don't have babies, though, you may find that you suddenly don't spend as much time with them as you used to. It isn't anything about you or them, it is just that many people who don't have babies feel like they can't relate to you anymore. You are talking about milestones in your pregnancy, or in your child's development, and they are talking about a guy they met last night. Your vocabulary changes and your priorities change. You will more than likely meet other moms and parents that you may start hanging out with, and will see less and less of your non-baby friends.

Living Arrangements: If you live in a one bedroom apartment, you may find things get a little cramped going into the toddler years. Although babies start out small, after a few years they demand more space. It's important to keep an open mind about your options and find a larger place to live. It isn't a decision you need to make right away, but it is nice to be able to put together a nursery for your baby. However, nurseries aren't important. All that is important is that your baby has a safe, warm environment in which to thrive. They will not remember that their first room wasn't painted with ducklings and teddy bears. They won't remember that you struggled with space issues. They will remember they always felt loved, safe, and secure. On the plus side, a small apartment will be easier to be made "baby safe."

Life Plans: Another facet of life to consider before deciding when to start trying to conceive is to figure out what your life plan is. Where do you want to be in five years? Ten years? Make a list of your future goals and acknowledge how raising a child may affect them. It's not impossible to have a career and a baby at the same time, but sometimes the two can clash. Climbing the corporate ladder with a baby on your knee might be too demanding and overwhelming. At some point, you may have to prioritize which is more important of the two. Not to say you can't do both, but realistically you can't give one hundred percent to both. Will stepping down from corporate life be an option? Will you be able to be a stay at home mother for your child? Studies have shown that children who are raised in a family where one of the parents is always at home have a higher sense of responsibility and independence. Not only that, but they also stay out of trouble more often, and children with a parent at home graduate from high school and college at a higher rate than children who are "latch key" kids or in daycare at an early age. Even if you want to return to work, your husband could stay home. Figure out how you could accomplish this before getting pregnant—save up money so you can be at home during your child's most formative years, or find a way to make money at home. They are only small for a short period of time; they need you there with them while they are learning what it means to be a human child.

Lastly, be patient. Sometimes there is a sense of urgency and women expect they will get pregnant right away. This is not usually the case. The average couple takes about four months to conceive. Getting pregnant is a journey, and for a small population, it's a battle. Be prepared and persevere.

How Hard is it to Get Pregnant?

After you have considered all the possibilities and implications, you've made the decision to have a baby. Now it's just a matter of getting pregnant, right? Unfortunately, it's not as easy as all those unexpected pregnancies you hear about want you to think. Your health, your age, your weight, and even how long you have been trying are all factors in your conception.

On average, it takes a healthy couple in their mid-twenties four months to get pregnant. Within the first three months, forty percent of couples succeed, and after six months, seventy percent succeed. Eighty-five percent of couples conceive by the end of the first year. Less than ten percent of couples are eventually diagnosed with infertility and seek medical help.

Each ovulatory cycle, there is a fifteen to twenty-five percent chance that the sperm will fertilize the egg. A woman's fertility peaks at about twenty-four-years old and falls after the age of thirty. Don't let this discourage you. There are many things you can do to increase your fertility and have a successful pregnancy, and not all women are alike.

Scheduling a Preconception Visit

Whether this is your first baby or your fifth, consulting with your caregiver prior to trying to conceive will lead to a healthier pregnancy. Your caregiver will be able to uncover any health problems or other issues that will make trying to get pregnant easier and less stressful for you.

Your reproductive history is very important to discuss. Anything unusual in previous Pap smear tests, pregnancies, or your menstrual history will be brought up. Based on both your family history and the father's family history, you can find out if genetic testing is necessary. It is also suggested that you are up to date on all of your immunizations before you conceive. Additionally, if there are any medications you're currently taking find out how safe the medications are during pregnancy. If they are not considered safe during pregnancy, your doctor can prescribe different forms of the same medication or have you stop taking them until after delivery. It all depends on risk versus reward.

Although you can buy prenatal vitamins over the counter, ask your caregiver for either a prescription or a recommendation of a favorite brand. Prenatal vitamins are vital even before you get pregnant because folic acid is extremely important. You need a supplement with at least 400mcg before conception and at least 800 mcg after conception.

It's best to schedule the preconception appointment about three months before you begin trying to conceive. This gives you time to make any lifestyle, dietary, or environmental changes you need to make.

Genetic Counseling

Your doctor may refer you to a genetic counselor for a variety of reasons, such as if your maternal age is thirty-five years or older, you or the father have a strong family history of a genetic condition or chromosomal abnormality, or you've had a previous pregnancy with a birth defect.

During the consultation, your genetic risks will be discussed or ruled out. Through testing, they can find out if you are at risk for having a child with cystic fibrosis, Huntington's disease, phenylketonuria, Downs' syndrome, sickle-cell anemia, Tay-Sachs disease, Spina bifida, muscular dystrophy or mental retardation. After the findings, they will offer supportive counseling to interpret the data with you and analyze your options.

Connecting with Other Women

Trying to conceive can be stressful, especially when you feel like you're alone in your efforts. Reaching out to other women online can be a great support system. Real women across the country are going through the same waiting game as you are.

There are many different online forums where you can make an account and connect with other women. To name a few: pregnancy.about.com, babycenter.com, babybump.com, JustMommies.com, Cafemom.com, and themommyplaybook.com. Each forum has different categories you can choose to join. Some have due date groups, some have trying to conceive forums, and some have pregnancy loss groups. Find the groups that work for you and join in on the conversation. You can find answers to the most frequently asked questions, get answers to your questions, share your victories and your worries, and meet new friends. These forums are especially helpful if you don't have friends or family who have babies, or if you are not comfortable sharing intimate details with friends or family.

You will be surprised by how much detail you will provide on a forum. With anonymity, you are able to ask questions, embarrassing and personal or not, and get real world answers. You may not always agree with other people's opinions, whether researched or not, but they are a great resource while you're trying to conceive and even while raising a child. A word of warning for those who are new to pregnancy forums: Women who are pregnant are often filled with a jumble of hormones and can tend to become easily irate about the most innocuous-seeming post. Fights do break out, and you will find that the most flammable fodder is found in posts about breast milk versus formula, to circumcise or not to circumcise, and whether to vaccinate or not. This isn't only due to hormones, but to some people's inability to understand someone else's point of view while not agreeing with them. They believe that their beliefs are the only right beliefs, and they will do anything to convert the forum readers to their perspective. Sometimes, these discussions diminish into school yard brawls. Don't take anything said seriously. People will say things to you on the internet that they would never think to say to anyone out loud. This same anonymity that allows you to ask embarrassing questions, also allows people to change their personas and say things that they know should not be uttered in polite society. If you find yourself stressing over the discussions in the forums, then they have become more of a hindrance than a help, and you need to step away from them for a time.

Chapter 2: Fertility

How to Boost Your Fertility

Fertility and lifestyle generally go hand-in-hand, so if you want to boost your chances of getting pregnant there are a few personal factors you should look at first. You need to look at how healthy you are and make any changes necessary to increase your healthiness. You should also learn more about how your body works, and how your cycle works. It's helpful to stop smoking and drinking. You should also cut down on the amount of caffeine you ingest. Also, remember that if your sex life becomes too regimented, you may find that sex could become too boring and routine. To help your conception, don't forget to have sex spontaneously. You should also try to reduce your stress levels as much as possible. And remember, it isn't just *your* health and lifestyle choices that affect your chances of conceiving, but that of the father as well.

Being significantly overweight or underweight can hurt the possibility of conception. For women, being overweight is defined as having a body mass index (BMI) higher than 25. Underweight women have a BMI of 18.4 or less. The goal is to fall within the normal range of 18.5 to 24.9. However, if you are considered "obese," don't let that deter you. You can still conceive. It may take you longer than other women, and it may not. Just because you are overweight doesn't mean you are unable to become a mother. The crash diet you may attempt prior to trying to conceive (TTC) could have a more adverse effect on your health and ability to conceive than your current weight does. If you do decide to lose weight before you TTC, change your lifestyle instead. Learn to eat better, learn how to cook fresh foods and avoid processed, chemically-created foods. Exercise more each day—start by walking a bit at a time and aim for thirty minutes a day. Remember that the thirty minutes don't have to be done all at one time.

Knowing your cycle will help you conceive. After a few months of tracking your cycle, you may be able to pinpoint the day you will most likely ovulate. Most women, but not all, ovulate about fourteen days before their next cycle begins. Becoming familiar with your rhythm will help you catch your most fertile times. Learn more about tracking your cycle in IRREGULAR CYCLES

IF YOUR CYCLES are not 28 to 35 days in length, the first thing you need to do is analyze your lifestyle. Is there anything that you may be doing to jeopardize conception? If you have already changed your habits to boost your fertility, you should begin to track your ovulation, which is a more in-depth process than simply charting your cycle. This is covered in the next chapter. However, if you do not have a regular monthly cycle, and instead have a period every few months, you may have polycystic ovary syndrome (PCOS), which can negatively affect fertility. If you think you may have PCOS, mention it to your caregiver. They can help by giving you fertility aids to increase your chances of ovulation.

Chapter 3: Tracking Your Ovulation.

Smoking can negatively affect fertility. If you smoke, stop. Cigarettes contain more than 700 different chemicals, many of which are poisonous to humans. Toxins from cigarettes are known to damage a woman's eggs and reproductive organs. Quitting often improves a woman's chances of getting pregnant, reducing the TTC period by up to two months.

It's debated how much alcohol and caffeine really affects fertility, but moderation is the key. If you are prone to partying, drink alcohol daily, or are a coffee addict, it's best to reduce your consumption to reasonable levels. When you do become pregnant, any alcohol habit should be kicked completely to prevent defects, such as fetal alcohol syndrome, and caffeine should be cut down to one cup a day. If you do have a drinking problem, however, it's best to seek treatment before you TTC.

Stress is not only a mood killer, but it is also a fertility suppressor. It can be difficult and patronizing when someone says, after months of TTC, "Relax, it will happen when it happens." However, there are a lot of benefits in not being too serious about getting pregnant. Keep it sexy and fun in the bedroom and don't turn it into an equation. While nearly everyone loves to have sex, if you make it too regimented or too important, you can kill the mood. Spontaneous sex can also boost fertility. Not only are you having fun and being intimate together, but the more often you have sex, the higher the probability you will catch the egg and become pregnant. Not only that, but spontaneous sex helps you relieve stress.

Now that you've taken a look at yourself, you should consider your partner and his habits. If he smokes, drinks, or uses drugs or steroids, he could be affecting the count and motility of his sperm. Just like a woman, he needs to keep his stress levels low, eat well, and exercise in moderation. Check out what type of underwear he uses as well, as tighty whiteys (briefs) can overheat his scrotum, impairing his sperm production. If he spends a lot of time in a hot tub, he could also be overheating his scrotum. See if he is willing to change his underwear habits from briefs to boxers. He could also sleep in the nude or not wear underwear at all. If he does use the hot tub often, ask that he limit the time in a hot tub during your fertile period. Another problem he could be introducing into the scenario that could affect his sperm production during your fertile cycle is his masturbatory habits. If he tends to masturbate often, he may not be able to keep up with his sperm production. Ask that he withhold from any sort of ejaculation until your fertile cycle, and then only if it will benefit you both.

When Are You Most Fertile?

A woman is most fertile beginning after the tenth day of her cycle. Some women ovulate on the fourteenth day of their cycle, some ovulate much later. The only real way to figure out your most fertile days is by tracking your cycle. The average menstrual cycle is 28 days long, so ovulation would fall right in the middle on cycle day 14. Typically, there is a 7 day "fertile window" that lasts from five days before ovulation until the day after (since the egg only has a 24 to 36 hour lifespan). The best time to have sex is right before ovulation. Once the egg "drops" and descends through the fallopian tube, the lower the chances are of it being fertilized. Most people do not realize that the egg is fertilized while it is still in the ovary or just beginning its descent through the fallopian tube. It does not become fertilized after it has reached your uterus. That being said, however, it is important to note that sperm can stay alive inside a woman for up to six days, so even if you have sex five days before ovulation, there is still a chance that your egg will be fertilized.

Possible Fertility Issues

If you are a healthy couple who are in their twenties, and have been TTC for a year, make an appointment with a fertility specialist or ask your caregiver to refer you to one. If you are a healthy couple in your thirties and have been TTC for six months with no success, make an appointment with a fertility specialist. You may need to be referred, so speak to your obstetrician/gynecologist (OB/GYN) or midwife first. Similar to your preconception visit, you will be asked questions about your sexual and gynecological history, in order to rule out possible causes.

Irregular Cycles

If your cycles are not 28 to 35 days in length, the first thing you need to do is analyze your lifestyle. Is there anything that you may be doing to jeopardize conception? If you have already changed your habits to boost your fertility, you should begin to track your ovulation, which is a more in-depth process than simply charting your cycle. This is covered in the next chapter. However, if you do not have a regular monthly cycle, and instead have a period every few months, you may have polycystic ovary syndrome (PCOS), which can negatively affect fertility. If you think you may have PCOS, mention it to your caregiver. They can help by giving you fertility aids to increase your chances of ovulation.

Chapter 3: Tracking Your Ovulation

Your Cycle

On average, a woman's menstrual cycle is 28 days long, but they can range anywhere from 21 to 35 days.

The first half of a woman's cycle (from day 1 to 14) is called the Follicular Phase. It begins on the first day of a woman's period, when hormone levels have dropped, signaling the body to shed the lining of the uterus. Bleeding typically lasts five days, although this can vary from woman to woman.

Once the menstruation is finished, the hypothalamus signals to the pituitary gland to produce follicle-stimulating hormone (FSH) and luteinizing hormone (LH). FSH encourages the maturation of an egg in the developing follicles. These follicles are located in your ovaries and have been there since you were a baby in your mother's womb. Each month, an egg is matured and released from a follicle (out of millions) and released. To release the eggs, FSH and LH must be present. To begin the process, the follicles start to secrete estrogen, which stimulates the production of gonadotropin-releasing hormone (GnRH), which in turn, increases the production of LH. The rising estrogen levels also stimulate the endometrium (lining) of the uterus to be built back up. This lining is what is shed during menstruation, and is built up again each month to provide a cozy, safe haven for your possibly fertilized egg. Around day seven of your cycle, if you have the 28-day "normal" cycle, the dominant follicle has matured, and the others start to degenerate. Usually there only is only one egg, but in some cases (due to fertility drugs or natural reasons) there are more than one. If more than one egg drops and becomes fertilized, you will be pregnant with fraternal multiples. Fraternal multiples happen when more than one egg is fertilized by the man's sperm. Maternal multiples are created when one egg is fertilized by the male, but then the egg splits into two separate babies. Maternal multiples are more similar in appearance than fraternal multiples.

Mid-cycle, your estrogen levels are at their highest, causing a LH surge as well as a FSH surge. Within 24-48 hours of the peaking of these two hormones, the follicle ruptures and releases the matured egg. This is ovulation. Some women report feeling a twinge in one side of their body, near one of their ovaries, around this time and are sure they are feeling the release of the egg.

The release of the egg signifies the start of the latter phase of the menstrual cycle called the Luteal Phase. As the egg begins its travels down the fallopian tubes, FSH and LH finish up their run by transforming the remains of the dominant follicle into the corpus luteum. The corpus luteum secretes progesterone, which is thought to act as an indicator for sperm and will help lead the sperm to the egg. The egg only has a lifespan of 24 to 36 hours, which is why a woman is most fertile 3-4 days before she ovulates up until only one day after. After approximately fourteen days, if the egg enters the uterus without being fertilized, it degenerates and the uterine lining begins to shed, starting the cycle once again.

However, if implantation does occur, the blastocyst (the fertilized egg) starts secreting the hormone called human chorionic gonadotropin (hCG, or the pregnancy hormone), which signals to the corpus luteum to continue its production of progesterone. The progesterone helps your uterus retain its lining, giving the blastocyst safe haven, and allowing the blastocyst to implant itself into the lining. Some women report feeling a slight cramping period mid-cycle which they think may be related to implantation. Still others report a brief spotting during this time, which is often referred to as implantation bleeding.

The length of the luteal phase is most consistent among women, lasting approximately fourteen days. When a woman has a luteal phase shorter than ten days, it is not usually long enough to sustain a pregnancy, and she should speak to her doctor immediately.

Overview: Ovulation Tracking Methods

On average, a woman's cycle is 28 days long and she ovulates on day 14. However, a lot of women don't, even if their cycle is 28 days long. Thankfully, there are a variety of methods used to track ovulation from the use of ovulation prediction kits or fertility monitors to taking your temperature and charting it daily to checking your cervical mucus and cervical position.

Ovulation Predictor Kit (OPK)

An Ovulation Prediction Kit (OPK) is used to determine when a woman may ovulate. The OPKs operate similarly to pregnancy tests. Either a woman can urinate on the test stick or place it in a cup of urine for a few seconds. An OPK works by detecting the LH surge that occurs 24-36 hours before a woman ovulates. Unlike a pregnancy test, these test strips are best used between 11am and 8pm—not the first morning urine. These are the hours in which the LH surge is most likely to occur. Also, unlike a pregnancy test, two lines do not necessarily mean a woman is having her surge. The test line must be darker than the control line. These are best taken starting day ten of your cycle. Each box contains between five to nine test sticks, giving you more than enough to catch your ovulation if you test daily.

Compared to other methods of detecting ovulation, OPKs are extremely convenient. They are available at most supermarkets or drugstores and don't require a daily commitment. However, it's important to remember that OPKs don't test for actual ovulation. Occasionally, a woman has her LH surge, but fails to release an egg. Sometimes, the OPK misses the LH surge, as it is only in the urine for six hours. If you test before or after that time is up, nothing will detect the LH surge. OPKs also don't indicate whether a woman's cervical mucus is fertile or if it is the best environment for sperm to travel through. Because of this, OPKs are best when used in addition to other methods.

OPKs can get pricey. They can range from $10 to $50 or more a pack. There are cheaper OPKs available online than you can find at the supermarket. They are usually no-nonsense brands, but can detect the surge just as well as name brands found at the store. They usually come in bulk and are approximately $1.00 a test.

What is a Fertility Monitor?

OPKs are great for determining two peak fertility days. However, there are now fertility monitors on the market that can identify up to six fertile days by tracking two hormones: luteinizing hormone and estrogen. These are fertility monitors.

The fertility monitor is started on the first day of your cycle, which means on the first day of bleeding. At this time, all you normally need to do is press a button to indicate your period has started. You press this button daily at the around the same time. Most monitors calculate the day based on when you pressed the button and allow you to press it the next day within a certain time frame of that first push. For instance, if you pushed the button at eight in the morning on day one of your cycle, you should press it within three hours of that time (either before eight or after eight) for the monitor to calculate that a day has passed. If you miss this time, then you've missed a day. The fertility monitor will usually have you start peeing on a stick (POAS) on the sixth day of your cycle during your first cycle using the monitor, but during the second cycle, it will have you start POAS later, since it has a pretty good idea on when you will most likely detect your LH surge. Simply hold the test stick in the urine stream, the data will be collected and interpreted by the monitor. When you first POAS, it will indicate whether you are at low fertility or high fertility. If it indicates high fertility then that is the best time to start having sex. When it indicates peak fertility, that means that your LH surge was detected and ovulation is imminent. It will usually register peak fertility for up to three days after the LH surge is detected. Then it will show one more day of high fertility and then low fertility. Once it has detected a few days of low fertility, it will stop having your POAS. At this point, you will just push a button daily until your period starts and you begin the cycle again, or you get a positive pregnancy test.

Fertility monitors vary in price, and they are the most expensive of all fertility prediction methods. Clearblue Easy offers theirs for around $200. Lady-Comp Fertility Monitor sells for nearly $500. But for women who have already tried other methods of predicting ovulation unsuccessfully, this may be a good option for them. You can find them used, which can be money-saving, and while the brands don't advocate using a used monitor, it doesn't mean you can't. If you do purchase a used one, make sure you clean the outside well—the manual tells you how to clean it—to ensure that any urine left on the device is gone. You don't pee on the machine, but on a stick, so it isn't as though you will be receiving a urine soaked monitor. It's completely up to everyone's comfort level, however. If you just can't bring yourself to handle something that someone else handled or inserted a urine-soaked stick into, don't buy it used. If you plan to have more than one child, or if you've already bought months' and months' worth of OPKs than the price of the machine could be beneficial. After the initial purchase of the machine, you only need to purchase the sticks.

What is BBT Charting?

Basal body temperature (BBT) is the lowest temperature the body reaches, usually during sleep. It is best measured immediately after waking, before even getting out of bed or drinking water.

Charting your basal body temperature is a fail-proof method used to determine when a woman ovulates. Unlike ovulation predictor kits, it will show you exactly what day you ovulate on, or if you have even ovulated at all, when done correctly. However, unlike OPKs and monitors, it will take a few months before you can accurately predict when you are going to ovulate.

To start BBT charting, you need to buy the proper thermometer. For BBT charting, accuracy is key, so the thermometer needs to be able to register $1/10^{th}$ of a degree. There are some thermometers that are accurate to $1/100^{th}$ of a degree; these are nice, but they're not necessary. If you are without a thermometer at home, a BBT thermometer can easily be purchased for about $10 at any grocery or convenience store (like Pathmark or Walgreens). Just be sure that it says it is a basal body temperature thermometer before purchasing one.

In addition to the thermometer, you will need a place to keep track of your temperature readings. The best online charting site is FertilityFriend.com, which, though there is a paid member feature, it is free to use. Simply sign up and input the data daily. There is even an app now available for smart phone users. This is great for visualization. If you do not have access to the internet, you can create your own daily chart. This chart will be where you write your temperature, but it can also contain other pertinent information, such as when you had sex, if you had a headache that day, what your cervical mucus or cervical position was like, whether you felt crampy, started your period, or tested positive. This method is nice, because when you do test positive for pregnancy, you can usually pinpoint your exact ovulation day, which can make your due date more accurate.

For the best BBT reading, take your temperature first thing in the morning when you wake up before you even get out of bed. Make sure you've had at least five consecutive hours of sleep and that you're consistent about your wake up time (variations of 30 minutes are okay). For example, if you take your temperature at eight every morning, any earlier than 7:30 or later than 8:30 will create errors in the data.

The best time to start charting your BBT is on the first day of your cycle. After a few months of experience with charting, you may find that you skip the first couple days of your cycle because this data is less important, and you already have an idea of when you ovulate.

During the follicular phase of your cycle (approximately the first 14 days), your temperature will vary day to day. It may go up and down, or it may only vary by 0.1 degrees. These are usually the lowest temperatures you will see during your cycle.

Right before ovulation, typically on day 14 or 15 (in a 28 day cycle), you will notice a drop in your temperature. Sometimes, because the drop is slight, this pattern is only noticeable after several months of temping. With other charts, it may be more obvious. Either way, this sudden drop in temperature is usually caused by your LH surge. The day after this drop, your temperature should increase by at least 0.4 degrees. This signifies that ovulation has occurred. If your BBT has not increased by at least 0.4 degrees one cycle, don't panic. Even a healthy, fertile woman experiences annovulatory (cycles in which ovulation does not occur) cycles occasionally. If it is consistent, it is best to speak to a fertility specialist. This peak in temperature signifies the start of the luteal phase. Your BBT will stay elevated until approximately 10 or 11 days past ovulation (DPO) (for some women, temperatures stay elevated until menses occurs). Should temperatures stay elevated and your period has not start as usual, this could mean you have become pregnant.

Sometimes, women experience what is called an "implantation dip" anytime between 5 DPO and 10 DPO. They find that their temperature dips significantly for one day and then rises again. This does not occur for all pregnancies, nor does it always mean a pregnancy has occurred.

After charting for a few cycles, hopefully you will start to notice a pattern. Most women have a biphasic pattern. During the follicular phase, temperatures are in a lower range, followed by a higher range during the luteal phase. Usually, you will ovulate around the same cycle day each cycle. So you can learn to anticipate and plan to have sex with your partner on the days leading up to ovulation.

Charting can be a huge aid to your caregiver, should you experience trouble getting pregnant. It can also help your caregiver spot any potential problems that may be preventing you from getting pregnant. As well, it can help your caregiver better predicate your estimated due date (EDD).

Analyzing Cervical Mucus

Cervical mucus (CM) is produced by the hormone estrogen and is secreted from the cervix. It is an essential aspect of fertility because it is the mode of transportation the sperm uses to get to the egg. Cervical mucus nourishes the sperm for up to five days (although some claim longer) and protects it from the acidity of the vagina. The consistency of your cervical mucus changes based upon the hormones your body is releasing during certain times in your cycle. By tracking cervical fluid, a woman can determine when she is most fertile.

To check your cervical mucus, insert your finger (make sure it's washed and dried well) into your vagina and get it as close as you can to the cervix. The best positions for this are sitting on the toilet or standing with one leg up on the edge of the tub. As you reach in, usually with your index finger, you will need to feel around for your cervix. Most women have no idea what they are touching down there, so don't be upset if you can't figure out what is what the first time you try. The farther up you are able to go, the closer to your cervix you are, and the more likely you are to get the mucus from the "source." Circle your finger around to collect a little bit of the mucus, and then remove your finger to analyze the mucus. Analyze the mucus by rubbing your finger and your thumb together. Do not check your cervical mucus after sex, though, as sperm, sexual stimulation, and personal lubricants will all affect your observations.

Once you have located your cervix, and you are more comfortable with your body, you can also try to collect as pure a sample of mucus as possible by inserting two fingers and gently pressing the cervix. This will allow the cervix to release mucus and you will be able to "scoop" it up and check it out.

Typically, right after your period you will find that the mucus is either dry or sticky. This means you are not currently fertile.

About a week before ovulation, you may notice that your mucus has a watery, tacky consistency which is usually infertile, but it could mean that your body is gearing up for ovulation. It may vary in color, either yellowish or white, and is usually opaque. This kind of mucus has no stretch to it. This means that if you put your thumb and finger together and then gently pull them apart, the mucus just stays on either finger and does not stay connected.

Wet or watery cervical mucus may mean ovulation is coming, and it is considered fertile mucus. It is generally clear, but may have a cloudy or white color to it. Watery cervical mucus has more of a stretch to it. Some women have even noted that it has a sweeter smell compared to non-fertile mucus.

Cervical mucus with a raw egg white consistency is the most fertile and indicates the best time to have intercourse. It is pliable and stretchy. It is the only kind of cervical mucus you can stretch between your thumb and forefinger. Some women never experience this kind of cervical mucus, so don't be alarmed or think you are infertile if you never notice it during your cycle. However, you will find that the more you check your mucus, the better you are at deciphering its meaning and consistency.

Creamy cervical mucus may resemble paste or it may be clumpy. This is non-fertile mucus and typically appears after your period or after ovulation.

Knowing how to check your cervical mucus can help you understand when the best time for intercourse will be. If you detect watery mucus, start having sex as often as possible. The best type of mucus for ovulation prediction, however, is egg white CM. This CM is most hospitable to sperm and helps the sperm swim up through the cervix, into the uterus, and up through the fallopian tubes. There are ways to increase your cervical mucus. For instance, taking guaifenesin in the days leading up to ovulation can help increase the amount of CM being released. Guaifenesin is the active ingredient in expectorants like Robitussin. Be sure that if you choose to use an expectorant that the only active ingredient is guaifenesin, as other ingredients may have the opposite effect. You should take two teaspoons (200 mg) of guaifenesin three times a day in the five days leading up to ovulation and on the day of ovulation. This will help increase the amount of CM released. As well, make sure you drink one eight-ounce glass of water with each dose. Another way to help your body release CM is by drinking plenty of water. The more hydrated you are, the more hydrated your CM will be.

Checking Your Cervical Position

Once you have figured out where your cervix is, and if you are checking your CM daily anyway, you can start to chart what position and texture your cervix is in every day. Your CM information and your cervical position can be added to your BBT chart as well. Before inserting your fingers into your vagina, make sure that they are as clean as possible, as you don't want to introduce any bacteria into your system.

Using the same position that you use to check CM, insert your fingers into your vagina. You will notice that the inside of your vagina is soft and pliable, but the further you reach in, you will find a spot that is firmer, rounder, and may feel like it has a dimple. This is probably your cervix. The texture and position of your cervix changes not only daily, but also during the day, so choose a time and stick to it. If the cervix feels firm, like the tip of your nose then you are probably not fertile. If it feels soft, like your lips, then you may be fertile. As well, you will find that the depth of the cervix changes (its position). If you find that it high and soft, and the dimple feels open, than ovulation is imminent.

If you start feeling for your cervix when you know you are not fertile, it will be easier to find. During menstruation it is very low and open to allow the uterine lining to shed. As you approach ovulation, your cervix rises, becomes softer in texture and the opening feels larger. If you haven't been pregnant before, the opening may be harder to detect. When you are no longer ovulating, the cervix closes, moves down, and becomes a harder texture.

The first few times you check your cervix, you may not really understand what you are feeling. With practice comes understanding and with understanding comes empowerment. Knowing how your body works and understanding the amazing process of your fertility, can give you a feeling of control over your fertility. Don't let social stigma stop you from experimenting with your body. Many women don't understand how our bodies work and are embarrassed by the thought of "messing around" down there. But don't worry about it. You aren't going to hurt yourself by exploring your reproductive cycles. Your husband pokes around in there, your doctor pokes around in there; why not explore it yourself?

Chapter 4: Making a Baby

The Best Sex Positions for Conception

Currently, there is no scientific research to support that any sex position is the best for conception, but that doesn't mean it isn't worth trying them all. It is believed that a woman's orgasm will help lubricate the sperms' approach and open up the cervix more to allow more sperm to come through. Also, the contractions caused by an orgasm can help sperm move up and into position.

Missionary position is a classic. With the man on top, the idea is that gravity does its work for you. The vagina is tilted downward, theoretically making an easier swim for the sperm. It's a very intimate position, allowing you to kiss each other and move freely the entire time during intercourse. This is the favored position, and most parents attest that it works the best.

From behind, also known as "Doggy Style," involves deeper penetration, getting him closer to the cervix and making it easier for the sperm to get to their goal. The man is usually in control in this position, which may intensify his orgasms as well. However, that doesn't mean the woman should just sit there. Rearing up a bit and pushing back during your partner's thrust can help both of you achieve orgasm.

Woman on top is a position that works against gravity, but it is can be more pleasurable for a woman.

After Sex Tricks

Although you may feel a bit silly doing them, there are some after sex tricks to increase the likelihood of getting pregnant.

First, right after intercourse, keep the penis inside for as long as possible to prevent leakage. Even as he exits, have him gently squeeze the labia to prevent his semen from dripping out. The more time the sperm has to swim to the cervix, the better.

To improve these chances even more, place a pillow or two under your hips and leave your hips elevated for fifteen to twenty minutes. This may also help the sperm on their journey.

My mom stood on her head for fifteen minutes to conceive me. I don't suggest this unless you are athletic and enjoy the position. It isn't essential, and is more than likely an "old wives tale" but if you've already tried everything else, it won't hurt to try it. However, you may want to warn your husband first.

Can I Use Lubrication?

Most lubricants are not sperm-friendly. Their pH value is too low and causes sperm death and decreases mobility. Stay away from KY Jelly, baby oils, and Vaseline. Even spit can have a negative effect on sperm. Thankfully, there are alternatives available for couples suffering from dryness.

PreSeed is scientifically proven to mimic fertile cervical mucus and has the perfect pH balance for sperm to stay nourished and get to the egg. The product comes with individually wrapped applicators that should be applied before sex, inserted close to the cervix, although it can also be applied directly to the penis as well.

Yes Baby is another sperm-friendly lubricant developed in the U.K. It is also certified organic. The packages come with two different formulas, one that is sperm-friendly (to be used during the fertile window) and one to restore vaginal pH after ovulation.

Conceive Plus advertises that they are the only sperm-friendly lubricant that has calcium and magnesium ions, which keep sperm nourished and healthy for their journey to the egg. They are available in single applicators or a multi-use tube.

A more natural alternative to market lubricants is coconut oil. It is probably the most inexpensive out of the sperm-friendly lubricants listed and is available at most health food stores. Even though it is solid, when it is applied to the hands and warmed, it dissolves into the skin and creates a very natural feel when applied to the genitals. There isn't much scientific evidence to back it up as a great method to conceive, but there are a lot of parents who swear by it.

How Can I Keep Sex from Feeling Like a Chore?

After trying for a few months, especially if you're charting and keeping track of ovulation, sex can begin to feel like a job. Your partner may even begin to feel performance anxiety. If you're beginning to feel this way towards each other and having a baby, it is time to refocus and rediscover romance in your relationship.

First, take a break from trying to conceive. Go on a date together that doesn't end up between the sheets. Enjoy each other. Be romantic. Push the stresses of baby-making from your mind and just be a couple together. You two could go on a picnic together, go dancing or even just curl up in bed and read a book together. If you still want to be intimate, but don't want to involve the pressure of sex, try finishing the night with some mutual masturbation. This will allow you to have the intimacy you crave, but take away the pressure of making a baby.

When it is time to have intercourse, change up the environment a bit. You don't always have to do it in your bed. Try the kitchen, or if you're flexible, the back seat of your car. You can make it exciting or romantic. If you go the romantic route, try playing some sweet music in the background, lighting some candles and bring out some warming massage oils. Before having sex, have a make-out session. How long has it been since you and your partner have just sat on a couch necking? It's probably been much longer than you actually thought.

Chapter 5: Eating To Get Pregnant

Diet and Fertility: What's the connection?

There haven't been a lot of studies to link food intake with fertility problems; however, a recent Harvard School of Public Health study was able to do just that. They followed a group of women over a long period of time, out of those women, some inevitably gave birth. While the study was not searching for diets and fertility, they were able to pinpoint areas in women who had problems getting pregnant and their diets that were similar. For instance, those who ate more "fast" carbohydrates like white bread, sugared soda, and white potatoes had a harder time getting pregnant. Those who ate carbohydrates from sources rich in fiber had higher rates of fertility. Not only that, but they also found that slowly digested carbohydrates coincided with a decrease in the chances of being diagnosed with gestational diabetes. This is good news for women all over the world who love carbohydrates. This means you don't have to completely cut them from your diet, instead choose carbohydrates that are slow to digest, have a low glycemic impact on your body, and are high in fiber. These not only keep you blood sugar lower, but they can improve your chances of getting pregnant. Choose carbohydrates from sources like whole grains, beans, fruits and vegetables. This is just one of the many foods that can help boost fertility.

What are fertility boosting foods?

Besides eating carbohydrates that are high in fiber and low in sugar and trans-fats, you can help boost your fertility by eating more plant-based proteins. The same Harvard study found that women who ate plant-based proteins more than animal-based proteins had an easier time conceiving a child and keeping it. Whole grains will give you a boost in B vitamins, vitamin E, and fiber. Eat fresh fruits and vegetables for vitamin C and helpful antioxidants. Lean meats and beans can give your body the protein, iron, and zinc it craves, while low-fat dairy products will also boost protein intake and calcium. Take DHA/Omega-3 supplements or eat canned light tuna, eggs, and salmon to help your baby's brain and nervous system develop. Omega-3 also helps prevent premature birth. Make sure your prenatal vitamin has at least 400 mcg of folic acid to help reduce the risk of having a baby with spinal cord and brain defects, but high is always better. You can also find foods that contain folic acid, mostly in fruits and vegetables.

Caffeine is also thought to interfere with conception. If you must drink coffee, try to limit your intake to no more than two five-ounce cups a day. Caffeine has the ability to cross the placenta and affect the baby, and has been thought to be a cause for some miscarriages.

Don't forget, however, that your health isn't the only factor in fertility. Look at the nutritional intake and health of your spouse. He may need to make some changes as well.

What Effect Does Diet Have On Male Fertility?

Make sure he isn't eating a lot of junk food. Not only does junk food make people fat and is terrible for the heart, but it also can impair the man's fertility. He should cut down on caffeine intake, as it can decrease his sperm count. Alcohol also serves this function, and should not be abused while you are trying to conceive. He should also avoid eating fish high in mercury. Fish that are high in mercury have a negative effect on both of your fertility factors. These fish include swordfish, tuna steak, and shark.

He can eat foods that help boost his sperm count, however. Foods like pumpkin seeds and oysters contain high amounts of zinc which can boost testosterone and sperm production. Pumpkin seeds are also a great source for Omega-3, which stimulates blood flow to his sex organs, which will improve their function. Other foods that are rich in omega-3s are almonds, fatty fish, and flaxseed. He should also eat more fresh fruits and vegetables to protect his sperm from cellular damage and keep them strong and fast. Vitamin A is important for a man's diet, as it helps prevent slow sperm movement and can be found in leafy greens, red peppers, apricots, and carrots. He can also consume pomegranate juice as it has been found to increase the sperms' quality and count in mice.

The Fertility Diet

The Fertility Diet is a book that was created from the Harvard study and contains steps to improve fertility and ovulation. Unlike other diets, this one is based on a scientific study and on scientific facts. The book can be purchased from any bookstore or online retailer. It was written by Jorge, E. Chavarro, MD, Walter C. Willet, MD, and Patrick J. Skerrett. The book states that it offers a diet plan that will improve your fertility and ovulation, offer a healthy start to your pregnancy, and one that is good for your body throughout your pregnancy and for the rest of your life.

The PCOS Diet

If you have been diagnosed with Polycystic Ovary Syndrome (PCOS), you may get information from your caregiver on diets that can improve your body's ability to ovulate; however, there are a few books out that contain information to help you understand the syndrome and give you the ability to reverse the effects through diet. One such book is *The PCOS Diet Plan: A Natural Approach to Health for Women with Polycystic Ovary Syndrome* by Hilary Wright, M.Ed., RD. The author is a registered dietitian who has worked as the Director of Nutrition Counseling for the Domar Center for Mind/Body Health at Boston IVF—a very successful fertility clinic. She is also a nutritionist for the Dana Farber Cancer Institute in Boston. The book will help you try to understand PCOS, reduce your weight, risk of heart disease, and diabetes. It gives you an in-depth diet plan, which includes a shopping guide and a guide for eating out. It will give you resources for support, pregnancy planning and a way to integrate the diet into your everyday life. It even has sample meal plans to get you started.

The Gluten Free Diet May Improve Male Fertility

Going gluten-free is a major movement in today's food intake community. Some people have undiagnosed celiac disease, which can cause infertility. Celiac disease makes your body react strongly to gluten, causing your body's immune system to attack the lining of your small intestines, which stops you from absorbing nutrients. Sadly, while the effect of celiac disease in women's fertility has undergone extensive study, studies on male infertility and celiac disease has been virtually ignored. However, a few studies have shown that men with celiac disease have poor sperm quality and low sperm count. If you are having trouble conceiving, ask your spouse to get checked for celiac disease. If celiac disease is the problem, switching to a gluten free diet can increase his fertility. However, if he doesn't have celiac disease, switching to a gluten free diet won't increase his fertility, though it may help him lose weight and feel better. If he does have celiac disease, he must switch to a gluten free diet and follow it strictly, for life.

Chapter 6: The Right Bodyweight

How does weight impact your ability to get pregnant?

A study conducted and published in *Fertility and Sterility* in 2004 showed that overweight women took twice as long to get pregnant. What is even more surprising, especially in our culture focused primarily on losing weight is that women with a BMI of 19 or lower showed to have the most trouble conceiving. They took four times as long as women in the normal range. This shows that being overweight *and* underweight can have an impact on your ability to achieve pregnancy.

If you are overweight and considering trying to conceive, change your lifestyle, eat more fresh fruits and vegetables, and exercise daily to lose the excess fat. If you are underweight, eat foods that are healthy and high in good fats. Look for diets to help you gain weight until you can achieve a good BMI.

What is the recommended BMI for maximum fertility?

There is no golden BMI number for maximum fertility; however, a mid-range BMI is the healthiest. Talk to your caregiver and find out where you stand, and whether or not you will need to gain or lose weight. Women who have a high BMI have less successful fertility treatments than people with a mid-range BMI. If you are diagnosed with infertility, you may need to lose or gain weight before undergoing any infertility treatments to enhance their success rates.

Chapter 7: Lifestyle Factors

Fertility and Alcohol

Some studies have shown that even women who drink as few as one to five alcoholic drinks a week take longer to get pregnant that those who do not drink at all. The more alcohol you drink, the lower your probability of getting pregnant. However, as is obvious from the large amount of babies born to couples who drink, don't let it fool you into thinking it will never happen for you. If you do have a drinking problem, though, you should join a rehabilitation program and quit drinking before you decide to become pregnant.

Alcohol consumption can adversely affect the reproductive cycle. Women who drink often or who are alcoholic can have an absence of periods, lack of ovulation, or a shortened or abnormal luteal phase. This lack of ovulation is called anovulation, and usually, the woman continues to have a period, but her ovaries do not produce an egg every month. A shortened or abnormal luteal phase will not give the fertilized egg the time it needs to implant securely and release hormones before menses begins. If you are having fertility problems, quit drinking as soon as possible.

Alcohol also affects the fertility of men. Men who drink may have abnormal liver function, which can trigger a rise in the hormone estrogen, which in turn, could interfere with how well his sperm develops. Also, alcohol can kill off sperm-generating cells in the man's testicles, which can drastically lower the man's sperm count. If the man drinks and has been told he has a low sperm count, he should quit drinking and be tested again in about four months.

How does smoking affect fertility?

If you are a smoker, you know that there seems to be nothing sweeter than that first drag of the first cigarette of the day. The dark call of nicotine winds through your mind at all hours of the day, and sometimes, the night. However, cigarettes are full of other surprises, and besides the drug nicotine that you are addicted to, you are also introducing over 4000 other chemicals into your system. Smoking not only causes a myriad of cancers, but smoking while pregnant can increase the risk of a premature birth, birth defects, low birth weight, and stillbirth. Even if you have a seemingly healthy baby, smoking while pregnant can more than double the risk of sudden infant death syndrome (SIDS).

But can't you smoke while you are TTC and quit when you get pregnant? You could, but you may be TTC longer than necessary, and you are still introducing toxins to your baby during a very critical time of growth. Smoking can lower the chance of getting pregnant by up to forty percent. A study done on mice demonstrated that nicotine can negatively affect the maturation of eggs, as well, the mice's eggs showed more chromosomal abnormalities than eggs of mice that were not exposed to nicotine. Smoking can even affect the rate at which you will become pregnant through in vitro fertilization (IVF). However, women who quit smoking for a year were found to take no longer to get pregnant than women who had never smoked. That's a giant leap and it shows that quitting smoking is one of the better lifestyle changes you can make to increase your chances of conceiving.

Stress

Stress effects physiology. High levels of stress have been shown to lower the immune system's response, increase the chances of heart disease and cancer. When you are stressed, your cycles may not be optimal; stress can even stop ovulation. Stress increases blood pressure as well, which can have a negative effect on how the baby grows. Stress can cause the baby to be underdeveloped, as the high blood pressure decreases the amount of blood going to the placenta. It can also slow and stall labor. If you are under high amounts of stress, find ways to relax. Take baths, take walks, take deep breaths or learn a meditation technique that can help you cope with stress.

Chapter 8: Natural Supplements

The Importance of Prenatal Vitamins

It's well known how important prenatal vitamins are during pregnancy. Growing a new life requires all the right tools, and usually diet is not diversified enough to get the full gamut of vitamins and minerals necessary. Not as many women are aware that they should begin taking prenatal vitamins three months before they even begin trying to conceive.

Significant nervous system development occurs within the first few weeks of pregnancy, often before a woman even realizes that she's pregnant. Having a deficiency in certain vitamins can be extremely detrimental to the growth of the baby. When searching for the right prenatal, sufficient doses of these key vitamins should be considered.

- Vitamin A—4,000 IU (international units)

- Folic Acid—800 – 1,000 mcg

- Vitamin D—200-400 IU

- Calcium—200-300 milligrams (mg)

- Vitamin C—85+ mcg

- Thiamin—1.4+ mg

- Riboflavin—1.4+ mg

- Vitamin B-6—2.6 mg

- Niacin (or B3)—18 mg

- Vitamin B12—4 mcg

- Vitamin E—15 mcg or 11 IU

- Zinc—11+ mg

- Iron—27-60 mg

If the prenatal vitamins do not have these minimums, either buy additional supplements or find a brand that does.

Vitamins for Him

Women aren't the only ones who should take vitamins to boost fertility. Men may also have deficiencies that could be affecting the quality and quantity of their sperm. Make sure that he also takes a daily multivitamin, not only when you are TTC, but also to maintain a healthy lifestyle. His daily vitamins should contain calcium, folic acid, vitamin C and D, and zinc.

Chapter 9: Gender Selection

The Shettles Method

The Shettles Method was created by Dr. Landrum Shettles. He based his method around the belief that the x and y sperm are different from each other. The book for this method is called, *How to Choose the Sex of Your Baby* by Dr. Shettles. He talks about the differences in the two sperm types, and how to use those differences while TTC to get pregnant with the sex of your choice. The book reports that there is eighty percent effectiveness when using his method. For those who have no idea what this difference is or what an x or y sperm even is: The woman's egg is an X chromosome. The male's sperm are either X or Y chromosomes. When an egg is fertilized by an X chromosomal sperm, they merge (XX) and become a girl. When an egg is fertilized by a Y chromosomal sperm, they merge (XY) and become a boy.

According to Shettles, girl sperm have longer lives, are slower, and are hardier than male sperm. Accordingly, if you want to have a girl, you have sex two to three days before you are going to ovulate, which will allow the female sperm to outlive the male sperm. He also suggests that women avoid having an orgasm if they want to have a girl, as the vagina's environment becomes less favorable for the X-bearing sperm. He also suggests you avoid positions, such as doggy style, that offer a deeper penetration. If you want to conceive a boy, he suggests positions such as doggy style, having an orgasm, and having sex as close to the day of ovulation as possible.

While many women swear that this method worked for them, scientific studies show that this method does not work and that it can, in fact, make it harder to get pregnant.

The Whelan Method

This method was developed by Elizabeth Whelan, Sc.D. and it is based on timing of intercourse. This method works best if you are charting your BBT. She suggests that if you want to have a boy, to have sex four to six days before your temperature is set to rise, and three to four days before ovulation for a girl. Her reported success rates are lower than Dr. Shettles' method; however, unlike Dr. Shettles, she did not base the study on her own studies, but rather that of 1300 women who were charting their temperatures, wrote what day they had sex and reported the outcome. The outcomes are about a fifty-seven percent success rate for girls and sixty-five percent success rates for boys.

The O + 12 Method

This method is for people who only want to conceive a girl. It is based on the timing of sex, dependent on when you will ovulate. The study was performed by a mother in New Zealand who had six sons while doing the Shettles method. This study suggests that if you want to have a girl, you should only have sex twelve hours after you have ovulated, hence the O (ovulation) plus 12 (twelve hours) in the title, and then you are not to have unprotected sex until you are no longer fertile. The non-scientific study that the creator orchestrated showed a ninety percent success rate. All of this being said, however, it is important to note that having sex after ovulation can actually decrease the chance of the egg being fertilized and may mean that you will take longer to get pregnant than if you tried any other method. If you are using this method and are having trouble conceiving, perhaps you should start looking into other methods.

The Ericsson Method

This method is the most scientific of the methods mentioned so far. The man's sperm is given to a fertility clinic, which then separates the x-bearing sperm from the y-bearing sperm. They inseminate the female with the batch of sperm that contain the most x- or y-bearing sperm. This process is about seventy-five percent effective for male babies and about seventy-two percent effective for female babies. It does not rely on IVF, and is applied through intrauterine insemination.

The most effective form of gender selection is done via IVF and is also the most expensive. The doctors use embryos as well as sperm. Once the gender of the embryo is apparent through genetic diagnosis, the egg or eggs are placed in the mother's womb. This form of gender selection is almost 100 percent accurate.

Eating to Conceive a Boy

Many studies have been done on which foods present the woman with a higher chance of conceiving one sex or another. If you want to have a boy, studies have shown that eating more of the following foods while TTC or even in early pregnancy, can help you have a boy.

Alkaline Foods: Y-bearing sperm supposedly live longer in alkaline environments, knowing which foods have a higher percent of alkaline can help:

- Cereals—a study done at the University of Exeter and Oxford, which followed several hundred pregnant women, determined that women who ate two bowls of cereal a day had a higher rate of having boys.

- Salty Foods—another study showed that women who ate more salty foods had a higher rate of boys. Avoid empty calories, and instead opt for foods like red meat, eggs, and beans, just add more salt than you normally would.

- Potassium—eating foods high in potassium is also another way to help you conceive a boy. Bananas, avocados, raisins, and nuts (among others) contain potassium and can be easily included in your diet.

- No Dairy—dairy products are thought to increase the acidity of the vaginal environment, so while you need calcium, find a different way to get your calcium if you are trying to conceive a boy. You can take supplements, buy foods with higher calcium content, or eat more spinach.

You can test your vaginal environment for acidity by using a pH testing kit. These can be found in health food stores or even at your local fish store.

Eating to Conceive a Girl

To change your acidity in the vagina towards a more girl friendly environment, eat foods that are high in acid like citric fruits. Your diet should be low in salt and potassium and high in calcium and magnesium. This diet would be pretty much the opposite of eating to conceive a boy.

Chinese Gender Chart

Chinese gender charts proliferate on the internet. They supposedly have ninety-nine percent accuracy in predicting what sex you will be having. You can use the calendar to decide which month(s) you will TTC for a certain gender. On a side note, it has not accurately predicted that all six of my babies would be girls. Based on the outcomes I have received, I find the accuracy to be more like seventy percent accurate. This chart is based on your age and the month you conceive to show what gender you will conceive or have conceived.

How to Increase the Likelihood of Twins

If you have a family history of twins, the likelihood is higher that you will have them. It does not matter if twins run in your husband's family, only if they run in yours. Twins are a maternal miracle. You either release two eggs simultaneously and they are fertilized by two sperm or you release one egg which is fertilized by one sperm and then splits. The first choice is the hereditary influence; if you have a maternal unit who had twins, then you may have inherited a gene that causes hyperovulation. Splitting of the egg, however, is completely by chance. There is no gene as yet known that stimulates an egg to split.

Another way to increase your chances is to gain weight. A study by the American College of Obstetrics and Gynecology (ACOG) found that the rise in multiple births correlated with the rise in obesity.

You may also wait until you are older to have twins. Women who conceive after the age of forty-five have shown to have a higher chance of having multiples.

Eat plenty of yams. The Yoruba tribe of West Africa has the highest rate of multiples in the entire world. Why? A study of the tribe showed that the mother's diet could have been the cause. The women of the Yoruba tribe eat a lot of yams.

Go to a fertility clinic. Couples who choose IVF to conceive often have multiple babies, this is because more than one egg is inserted into the uterus to increase the odds of at least one implanting. However, often more than one of the eggs implants.

Having a big family can also increase your chances of conceiving twins. The more kids a person has, the higher their chances of having twins in another pregnancy. There is no magic number of children that will allow twins to happen, so if you really want twins, you just have to keep trying.

Have a lot of sex while you are breastfeeding. While most people believe that breastfeeding is a foolproof method of birth control, this is often wrong. A woman can ovulate at any time during breastfeeding and lactating and many women find this out the hard way. However, one doctor claims that women who conceive while breastfeeding are nine times more likely to have twins than those who are not breastfeeding.

Chapter 10: Getting Pregnant with Ailments

What is infertility?

A healthy couple under the age of 34-years old should be able to fall pregnant within six months. For ages 35 and older, this time window expands to one year. If you have been trying longer, or are unable to sustain a pregnancy to full term, you should make an appointment with a fertility specialist or Reproductive Endocrinologist. Approximately 10% of couples in the United States suffer from infertility, but there are now many effective therapy options available.

How do I get pregnant with PCOS?

Polycystic ovary syndrome (PCOS) occurs when the ovaries produce too many androgens (male sex hormones), which may cause a woman to stop ovulating or cause her to ovulate in an inexact pattern. It is the most common cause of infertility. Once you are diagnosed by your caregiver, there are a variety of treatments available to you.

Natural treatments include regular exercise, healthy foods, and weight control. Moderate activity, such as walking, should be worked into your daily routine. In addition, it's important to eat a heart-healthy diet. Cut back on foods that are high in saturated fats and sugars and begin to incorporate an array of vegetables, fruits, nuts, beans and whole grains into your diet. Losing just ten pounds has shown to help balance hormones and regulate the menstrual cycle.

If lifestyle changes aren't enough to harmonize your hormone levels, your fertility specialist may prescribe medication. Although birth control pills and spironolactone, an androgen-lowering drug, are usually prescribed and are very successful at alleviating symptoms, they are not used if you are trying to get pregnant. Glucophage (Metformin), the leading treatment for women trying to conceive, is a diabetes medication that can help stabilize hormone levels and fertility. Clomiphene (Clomid), an ovulation-stimulating drug, is the most effective treatment by replicating estrogen in the body. Femera (Letrozole) does just the opposite as it actively suppresses the estrogen in your body, which signals the brain to produce FSH. If all oral therapies fail, there are a group of medications called injectable gonadotropins, which encourage a woman's eggs to mature for ovulation.

High Prolactin Levels

Prolactin is the hormone that causes milk production. High prolactin levels are usually present after a birth, staying elevated for at least four to six months if a woman decides to breastfeed. It stops the release of FSH and LH, acting as a natural form of birth control. However, there are other causes of high prolactin levels that could keep an otherwise healthy woman from getting pregnant.

Prolactinoma is the most common kind of pituitary tumor, and it over-stimulates the secretion of prolactin. Medication is most often used to treat it and restore normal pituitary function. Normally, dopamine prevents the secretion of prolactin. Drugs, such as bromocriptine or cabergoline, called "dopamine agonists" act similar to dopamine and help to shrink the tumor. If this is unsuccessful, surgery or even radiation are considered as further treatment.

After a Miscarriage

A miscarriage is a very difficult loss to endure, and every woman will mourn in her own time. It takes two to three months for a woman's body to recover, so she won't experience an increased risk of miscarriage for the next pregnancy. Some physicians may suggest waiting six months to a year, but once a woman has physically and emotionally recovered and has decided to try again there are a few things she may want to consider.

Although the chances of a recurring miscarriage are only 15%, it may be a good idea to consider consulting a specialist. If you have had two or more miscarriages, an illness that may affect your pregnancy, fertility issues, or are over the age of 35, it would be wise to speak with someone involved with genetics or reproductive endocrinology.

Worry can seep in quickly, and a woman with previous miscarriages may become overly concerned. Don't be shy to ask that your pregnancy be monitored closely. Most caregivers will be more than willing to do this. If you find that you're struggling emotionally, speak with your caregiver about referrals to a support group or counseling that can help.

Chapter 11: Holistic Methods

How can herbal medicines help me get pregnant?

There has not been a lot of research on this subject. While there have been small studies done on herbal supplements formulated for enhancing reproduction, there have not been enough to point at certain herbs and say, "This one works the best." Herbal supplements can be counterproductive or can interfere with other medications. However, some herbs can help not only with conception but with pregnancy.

Which herbal supplements are best?

With all of these herbs, unless otherwise specified, they should not be taken after ovulation has been confirmed, and especially after the pregnancy has been confirmed.

- Chaste tree berry, one of the main ingredients in many fertility blends, has been linked to fertility. Chaste tree berry has been found to possibly increase fertility and to regulate menstrual cycles.

- Black cohosh is said to stimulate egg production. However, black cohosh has also been used as a natural way to induce pregnancy loss, so if you decide to try it, be sure you have the information you need.

- Red clover can balance the function of your hormones and contains estrogen-like compounds, which can help promote the production of estrogen.

- Siberian ginseng also regulates hormones.

- Lady's mantle tones the cervix and regulates the menstrual cycle.

How does acupuncture aid fertility?

According to current research, acupuncture is theorized to trigger hormones and chemicals to aid fertility. There has not been a lot of research on acupuncture and infertility, but the little that has been gleaned from the small amount of research suggests that acupuncture can

- improve pregnancy rates during IVF treatments when the acupuncture is performed on the same day as the IVF

- increase blood flow to the uterus

- reduce stress and anxiety

- improve ovulation for women who have PCOS

- regulate the hormone that regulates ovulation

- and improve the man's sperm count and quality

The Benefit of Chiropractic

One study showed that women who were infertile and underwent chiropractic adjustments later became pregnant. Chiropractors suggest that when the body is out of balance and the spine is not aligned correctly, it does not allow the egg to be delivered to the uterus. They also suggest that the nerves that are connected to the reproductive system are also attached to the spine and any distortions in the spine can affect fertility. While this study was small, it could have big benefits. If you have had menstrual problems such as PCOS or have been diagnosed with endometriosis, trying chiropractic treatment could do more for you than any surgeries or drugs may. It doesn't hurt to try.

Feng Shui for Fertility

Not everyone is a believer in feng shui. However, it is not invasive, so it wouldn't hurt to try it. To increase your feng shui for fertility, display such things as open pomegranates, images or elephants (or statues) with their trunks relaxed, or pictures of babies in your home or bedroom. You can also have a feng shui consultant enter your home and find the weak areas in your house. Some suggest that you do not have a ceiling fan above your bed, and not to move your bed if you are trying to conceive. Also, it has been suggest that you have children jump on your bed as much as they like to energize and invite fertility.

Asian Bodywork for Fertility

Asian bodywork includes chi nei tsang, shiatsu, and tui na, and all of these try to bring the body into balance—to find that balance between yin and yang. The best way to find a method that is good for you is to visit specialists in all practices and choose the one that fits best with you and your beliefs. All techniques try to find areas that are out of balance for fertility, based upon their beliefs. Treatments range in price from thirty to one-hundred-fifty dollars, but some may offer free consultation.

Chapter 12: Fertility Medications

How do I determine if I need fertility medications?

Your fertility specialist will order various tests and procedures to determine if you are ovulating, and if there are any hormonal imbalances that can be corrected with medication.

- Blood tests will be run to check for certain hormone production, such as your levels of follicle stimulating hormone (FSH), luteinizing hormone (LH), prolactin, estrogen, and thyroid stimulating hormone (TSH).

- The Clomiphene Challenge Test analyzes how well your ovaries function, and how they respond to Clomid, a particular fertility medication. Blood will be drawn on the third day of your cycle and again on the fifth day (when you start taking Clomid). On the tenth day, blood will be drawn for the third time, and the results will help to determine how aggressive your treatment should be.

- An endometrial biopsy is performed to assess the quality of your uterine lining as well as to determine if you're ovulating or not. It's most often used for women with previous miscarriages or a short luteal phase.

- Hysterosalpingogram (HSG) is a procedure in which your doctor will inject a blue dye through your cervix into your uterus and trace its movements using an x-ray. The goal is to find out if there are any blockages in your fallopian tubes. This method is also used to map the contour of your uterus or see if you have any polyps, fibroids or other abnormalities that could be affecting your ability to get pregnant.

- A laparoscopy is a surgical procedure where anesthesia will be given so your doctor can check your reproductive organs for signs of scarring or endometriosis. This is usually performed after an HSG has come back abnormal.

- Pelvic ultrasounds are a non-invasive procedure that the doctor can use to determine the thickness of your uterine lining, whether or not your follicles are growing properly, and can also be used to identify cysts or fibroids.

- A hysteroscopy is a procedure in which the doctor will use a tiny scope (a thin tube with a camera on the end) to see the inside of your uterus. Although the camera cannot see your fallopian tubes, it does help to find abnormalities such as polyps or fibroids. It is usually used if an HSG comes back abnormal.

- A post-coital test involves both partners and evaluates the interaction between the cervical mucus and the sperm. You will be asked to have sex 24 hours prior to the exam, and then a sample of your cervical mucus will be taken. The sperm within the cervical mucus will be analyzed for its mobility, which will indicate if there are certain antibodies present in the mucus that could be impeding the sperms' progress.

- A semen analysis can be ordered for your partner. His sperm will be analyzed under a microscope for shape, count, appearance, and movement.

Clomid and other Fertility Drugs

Fertility drugs may be prescribed by your fertility specialist if they find that you are not ovulating on your own. These include Clomid, Metformin, Femera, and others.

- Clomiphene, also known as Clomid or Serophene, is a drug designed to stimulate ovulation. You take it for five consecutive days starting on day five of your menstrual cycle. It elevates your FSH levels, which encourages the maturation of eggs in the ovaries. Since it usually stimulates the development of multiple eggs, it is most often used in conjunction with assisted reproductive technology (ART).

- Glucophage, also known as Metformin, is a diabetes medication that is prescribed to women diagnosed with PCOS to lower insulin levels and regulate the menstrual cycle. It acts as an androgen suppressant when the ovaries and adrenal glands are over-producing the male hormone. It has a 45% success rate in women with PCOS and has shown to be more effective when used in conjunction with Clomid.

- Letrozole, also known as Femera, is most commonly used to treat early breast cancer, but can also be used as a fertility treatment because it lowers the amount of estrogen produced by the body. The result is similar to that of Clomid, encouraging the production of FSH and LH and increasing the number of mature eggs for ovulation. As a warning, there have been findings that women who took this drug while pregnant had a higher rate of birth defects. Although, there haven't been any documented cases of birth defects for women who took this medication before becoming pregnant, so it is still deemed safe as a fertility treatment.

- Follistim, Gonal-F, Bravelle and Fertinex are all follicle stimulating hormones (FSH), which regulates the maturation of a dominant egg in a woman's ovaries. It is usually used in combination with hCG. These subcutaneous injections can also be used by men to produce more healthy sperm. They are often prescribed to women who have been deemed Clomid-resistant or have PCOS. Women undergoing assisted reproductive technology procedures, such as IUI or IVF, may also take some form of FSH. A fertility specialist will use a sonogram to monitor follicle count size and growth every two to three days and will use the data to reevaluate dosage. These drugs cannot be prescribed for women with primary ovarian failure.

- Human Chorionic Gonadotropin (hCG), which can be given as Ovidrel, Novarel, Pregnyl or Profasi, is the hormone that supports FSH with the development of the egg in the ovaries. This version can be administered through injection and serves as a treatment for infertility in women and can increase sperm count in men. Occasionally, women using this medication may develop a condition called ovarian hyperstimulation syndrome (OHSS). This can be life-threatening, so it's important to communicate any side effects to the doctor administering the drug.

- Gonadotropin-releasing hormone (GnRH) antagonists, like Ganirelix, Antagon, and Cetrotide, is a synthetic protein that inhibits the production of follicle stimulating hormone (FSH) and luteinizing hormone (LH) at the pituitary gland. This is most often used for women undergoing in-vitro fertilization (IVF).

- Leuprolide, known more commonly as Lupron, Synarel, and Zoladex, is a gonadotropin-releasing hormone (GnRH) agonist. While GnRH antagonists stop the production of FSH, Leuprolide suppresses the pituitary and ovarian function. Because of its ability to lower estrogen levels, it's sometimes used to treat women with endometriosis.

- Human Menopausal Gonadotropin, also known as Menotropin, Pergonal, Humegon, Repronex, and Menopur, is a treatment for women who do not menstruate. Menotropin directly stimulates the ovaries to promote ovulation, unlike Clomid which acts on the pituitary gland. It has shown effectiveness in women with ovarian dysfunction, endometriosis and unexplained infertility. Women undergoing assisted reproductive technology (ART) may also be prescribed this drug.

- Heparin, also known as Hep-lock or Liquaemin, is an anticoagulant and helps to thin the blood, preventing clotting. Women suffering from multiple miscarriages may be prescribed this injectable medication because it has been successful in helping women carry a pregnancy to term. High levels of antiphospholipid antibodies in a woman's body have an increased risk of blood clots forming in the placenta, cutting off oxygen flow to the developing baby. Treatment is usually in conjunction with baby aspirin, and studies have shown that this can help a woman carry her pregnancy to full term.

Side Effects

Many drugs have potential side effects, especially if you are taking other prescription medications. Before starting any regimen of drugs, find out what the possible side effects are by asking your doctor or your pharmacist. You may find that the risk outweighs the rewards.

Chapter 13: Treatments for Infertility

What is Assisted Reproductive Technology (ART)?

Assisted Reproductive Technology (ART) includes fertility treatments that handle sperm and egg. Generally, these procedures involve removing eggs from a woman's ovaries and then fertilizing them with the male's sperm. Then, once the eggs are fertilized, they are placed into the woman's womb for maturation via In Vitro Fertilization. ART does not include insemination or medication to stimulate egg production unless the eggs are then going to be taken out of the ovaries. According to the Centers for Disease Control and Prevention, ART has been in use in the U.S. since 1981. With only 1% of all babies born in the U.S. conceived using this method, this procedure is not that common. It is expensive and time consuming; however, the use of ART has doubled in the last ten years. Many pregnancies that go to term using ART are multiple pregnancies. According to the most recent data that the CDC has published, the 47,090 live births resulting from this method in 2010 produced 61,564 babies.

Intracytoplasmic Sperm Injection (ICSI)

Intracytoplasmic Sperm Injection (ICSI) is a technique used in ART to treat couples with sperm-related infertility problems. It is the procedure in which the sperm is injected into the mature egg. After fertilization, the egg is placed into the woman's uterus or sometimes into the fallopian tube. The sperm is collected via masturbation, or if that is not a possibility, it is collected through a small incision in the testicle.

Intrauterine Insemination (IUI)

This form of fertility treatment is used when there are unexplained infertility problems, the man has a low sperm count or decreased sperm mobility or does not produce fertile sperm. It is also used if the cervix environment is hostile to sperm, i.e. there is not enough cervical mucus, the mucus is too thick, or there is scar tissue on the cervix. The procedure takes the man's sperm, or donated sperm, and using a catheter, the sperm is injected into the uterus. This will help increase the number of sperm that will make it up to the uterus and fallopian tubes to increase the chances of fertilization.

The procedure is performed using an ultrasound to monitor how big the egg follicles are to determine the timing of the IUI. Though it can be used without injected hormones, most women are asked to inject human Chorionic Gonadotropin (hCG) to stimulate the release of her eggs. They wash the semen to remove the sperm from the seminal fluid before injecting the sperm into the woman's uterus. After injection, a woman must undergo a two-week wait before finding out if she is indeed pregnant.

InVitro Fertilization (IVF)
IVF is the process in which fertilized eggs are surgically placed into the woman's uterus or fallopian tubes. There are two types of IVF treatments involving the fallopian tubes: the gamete intrafallopian transfer (GIFT) and the zygote intrafallopian transfer (ZIFT).

Gamete Intrafallopian Transfer (GIFT)
The GIFT procedure transfers the gametes (both the sperm and the eggs) into the fallopian tubes to allow the egg to be fertilized in the tube instead of in a laboratory. A laparoscopic procedure is used to place the gametes. This method is used in around 2% of all ART procedures in the U.S.

Zygote Intrafallopian Transfer (ZIFT)
The second fallopian procedure, ZIFT, transfers the fertilized eggs into the fallopian tube. It also involves a laparoscopic procedure and is used less often than the GIFT procedure—at about 1.5% of all ART procedures in the U.S.

Frozen Embryo Transfers (FET)
FET is the transfer of an embryo that was frozen immediately after it has been fertilized. This procedure can be used if the initial IVF treatment did not work, but more than a few eggs were fertilized in the initial treatment. A woman who will be having a frozen embryo placed into her uterus must undergo hormone therapy to make sure the uterine environment is optimal for implantation. First she must

suppress the pituitary gland by the use of the drug Lupron, which is injected daily for two weeks. She must also take the hormones progesterone and estrogen. These may be injections, pills, gels, or suppositories. First, the woman must take the estrogen supplements, and then once the uterine lining is thickened, they start taking the progesterone. This part of the cycle will start on a day that is chosen by the lab, to allow time for the frozen embryo to thaw before implantation. The progesterone is usually taken for five days, but can vary depending upon the lab and fertilization specialist.

Donor Egg or Embryo

Donor eggs may be used if the woman is over forty or has a high risk of having children with genetic disorders. The egg can be donated by a family friend, a family member, or an anonymous donor. When a donor is chosen, the woman and the donor will start taking Lupron. This will help sync up the cycles of both women. This is so that the donor woman ovulates when the woman who will receive the egg has an optimal uterine lining. Once the donor's eggs are mature, the doctor will remove them from her ovaries using a needle which is inserted through her vaginal wall and ultrasound is used to guide the needle. After the eggs are removed, the egg will be implanted using IVF.

Surrogacy/Gestational Carrier

An infertile couple may opt to have someone else carry their child. Maybe the woman never has optimal uterine lining or has a problem with her uterus that does not allow an egg to become implanted. Perhaps she has undergone a partial hysterectomy, and while she still produces eggs, she is not able to become pregnant. It may also be used if a woman cannot carry a baby to full term. Either way, the couple chooses a woman who will carry their child. The eggs are taken from the mother; the sperm is taken from the father. They are either fertilized in a lab or they may use the GIFT or ZIFT procedure. The gametes or the embryo are placed into the surrogate using IVF, and will carry the baby until it is born. After the baby is born, it is given to the parents. The parents usually pay for all medical bills, fertility treatments, and the birth. Sometimes, monetary compensation is also given to the surrogate for her time carrying the fetus.

Side Effects

Like any medical treatment, there may be side effects with any of these methods. Always discuss any possible side effects with your doctor before starting any medical treatment, so that you are aware of what problems, if any, may arise because of them. It is good to remember, as well, that the procedures are not foolproof. Many women must undergo a series of treatments before they become pregnant. There are also a lot of women who become pregnant with these procedures, and then have a miscarriage. Science is a wonderful tool, but it cannot make things happen one-hundred percent of the time.

Chapter 14: Pregnancy

Am I pregnant?

Every woman's body is different, but there are some common systems that point to pregnancy. Only you know what is normal for your body, and if you have been paying close attention to how your body reacts on the eve of menstruation, you can more easily assess changes as possible signs of pregnancy.

Keep in mind that most of these don't occur until HCG levels have reached quantities high enough to manifest with physical evidence.

- Backache: Although it's usually a later symptom, a backache can also signal pregnancy early on. Ligaments are loosening to prepare for the growth of the baby. This symptom will only worsen with weight gain and the shift in your center of gravity.

- Bloating and constipation: Due to the extra progesterone and an increase in water retention, you may experience a lot of bloating or even constipation early in pregnancy. Some women are bloated before menstruations also, so if this is a normal symptom for you, don't get too excited yet.

- Sore breasts: One of the most prevalent symptoms is sore breasts. Most women feel a bit tender leading up to menstruation, but if you are pregnant, it may be more pronounced, and you may even notice the darkening of your areolas.

- Food aversions or cravings: If you're finding that you're suddenly craving for strawberries or the thought of your usual cup of coffee turns your stomach, you may be pregnant. The surge of new hormones in your body can cause your food preferences to change (almost immediately, too).

- Fatigue: Making a baby is a lot of work, especially in the beginning, before the placenta takes over, which occurs around 12 weeks. Fatigue is often a response to the rising hormones as well as the amount of work your body is doing to create new life. The extent of the tiredness varies from woman to woman. You may find you are just as energetic as ever, or you may be so wiped out that you need a midday nap and are in bed by seven pm. Both are considered normal.

- Frequent urination: Most women don't experience frequent urination until the baby is larger, heavier, and sitting on their bladder. However, the increase in fluid levels in your body may have your kidneys (and your bladder) working overtime, even very early on.

- Headaches: The drastic changes in hormone levels may give you a headache. Keep in mind that ibuprofen is not safe to take during pregnancy, so if you suspect you are pregnant only take acetaminophen.

- Higher temperatures: During pregnancy, your basal body temperature will be elevated (you're a human incubator!) and you may even find that you have a very low grade fever during the day.

- Implantation spotting: Your period isn't due for another seven days, but you've had some brownish-red spotting for a few hours and then it stopped. This may be implantation bleeding which occurs when the egg burrows and attaches itself to the uterine wall, causing old blood to shed. This isn't a common symptom, so don't consciously look for it.

- Emotional changes: All the new hormones can be a lot to handle and can make a woman very emotional and moody. This is also a common symptom before menstruation.

- Morning sickness: Morning sickness is the most well-known pregnancy symptom, but this doesn't usually kick in until about six weeks along. It may manifest as nausea, or you may find yourself living off saltine crackers and ginger ale morning, noon, and night. It all has to do with your body and its reaction to the rising hormone levels.

- Shortness of breath: You may experience shortness of breath early in pregnancy. Increased blood flow delivering oxygen to the uterus can leave you feeling a little winded. Unfortunately, this feeling will only increase as the baby gets bigger and starts to put pressure on your lungs and diaphragm.

- Cramping: Unless you're one of the lucky few who escape it, all women experience cramping before or during their period, but it can also be a sign of pregnancy. Cramping may be from your uterus beginning to stretch to accommodate for the baby.

- Missed period: Perhaps one of the best indicators of pregnancy is a missed period. If your cycle is regular or you have been keeping track of it, and supposed cycle day one comes and goes with no menstruation, you might be pregnant.

The only way to truly tell if you are pregnant is to take a pregnancy test. We're lucky in this day and age, with pregnancy tests we can take at home that show results in three minutes or less. These tests are much more sensitive than tests of old, and you can even find some that can detect pregnancy six days before your period is due! Some women can get a positive result at only 8 or 9 DPO.

HCG Levels after Implantation

Human Chorionic Gonadotropin (hCG) is considered the "pregnancy hormone." It begins production after implantation and will double approximately every 36-72 hours.

On average, a pregnant woman may have an hCG level of 25 mIU two days before her missed period, although the range could be anywhere from 5-50 mIU. A day before her missed period, the average is closer to 50 mIU, with a range of 25-100 mIU. On the day of her missed period, those numbers increase again to 75 mIU on average, with a range from 50-100 mIU.

Pregnancy Tests

If you have any suspicion that you might be pregnant, you can either wait until after your missed period or go to the store to purchase a pregnancy test. There are currently a variety of different ones available, differing only slightly in price. Some are more sensitive than others. The best one is probably First Response Early Response, as it can detect hCG levels as low as 6.3 mIU, as early as five as or six days before your missed period.

Pregnancy tests are very easy to read. Two lines, even very faint, usually mean that pregnancy has been achieved. So, congratulations! Make sure you call your doctor to confirm and schedule your first prenatal visit.

Chapter 15: Summary

This book is meant to help you achieve conception, and to do so, we have covered nearly every topic about fertility, charting, medical and holistic methods, as well as behaviors to avoid before conception. However, it is only meant as a learning tool and not as the final solution. If you do not find the answer to your questions here, ask your doctor or midwife for more information. You can also try other books written on the subject, especially if you have specific fertility issue, as there are numerous books that will delve more deeply into that one subject.

Hopefully, this book has helped you better understand how your body works; knowing how your body works is the first step toward understanding fertilization. If you know the signs that your body gives you, it will make conception easier. Our bodies are miraculous things and every month it sends off signals that, if you are in tune with your cycle and your body, you will understand. You may begin feeling ovulation pain, where you had never noticed it before. Small things that you took for granted will become neon signs telling you that it is time to baby dance with your spouse. Take care of your body, learn from it, and it will help you in your journey towards motherhood.

Made in the USA
San Bernardino, CA
21 February 2018